KETO CHAFFLE

RECIPES

LOSE WEIGHT BY STIMULATING THE BRAIN AND
METABOLISM: A LOT OF RECIPES THAT
INTEGRATE YOUR KETOGENIC DIET
LOW CARB AND LOW BUDGET

CHRISTINE BUCKLEY

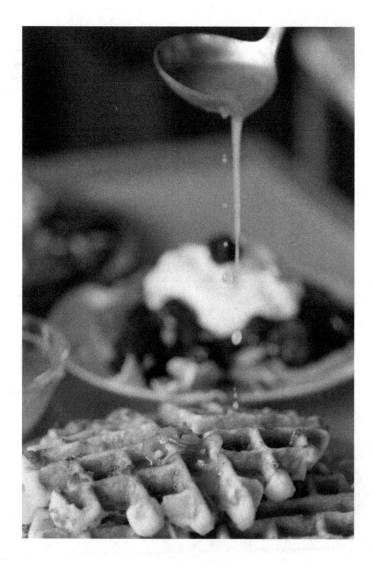

The information in the following pages is broadly considered a truthful and accurate account of facts and as such, any inattention, use, or misuse of the information in question by the reader will render any resulting actions solely under their purview. There are no scenarios in which the publisher or the original author of this work can be in any fashion deemed liable for any hardship or damages that may befall them after undertaking information described herein.

Additionally, the information in the following pages is intended only for informational purposes and should thus be thought of as universal. As befitting its nature, it is presented without assurance regarding its prolonged validity or interim quality. Trademarks that are mentioned are done without written consent and can in no way be considered an endorsement from the trademark holder.

TABLE OF CONTENTS

INTRODUCTION

Keto chaffles have taken the world by storm. Made with just two main ingredients, egg and butter, they can be prepared easily at home. You can eat them as sweet desserts, as a breakfast food, or as a snack. Chaffles are perfectly healthy foods that follow the

ketogenic diet recommendations.

They are high-fat, protein, and low-carbohydrate foods that can show the body how to use fat as an alternative source of fuel to produce energy and burn fat.

Thank you for downloading this book.

In this book, I will discuss chaffles and explain how they are different than waffles. I will ex- plain the various types of chaffles you can make easily at home. I will also go deep into the ketogenic diet and discuss its many advantages.

Finally, I will also share many mouth-watering Keto Chaffle recipes that are all easy to pre- pare. For each recipe, I will provide a list of ingredients and detailed step-by-step instructions. I am sure you will find this book very useful. Happy reading!

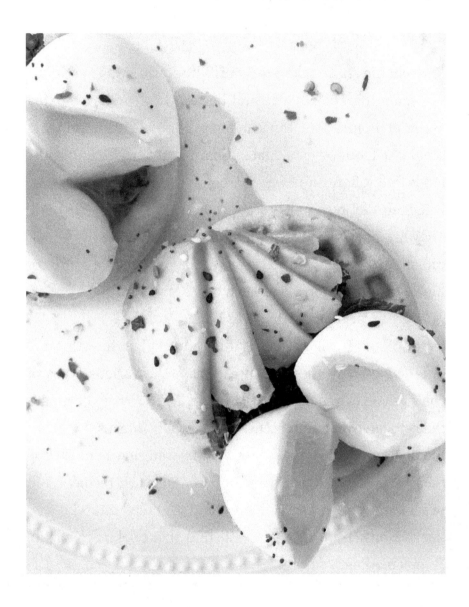

CHAPTER 1

FIRST OF ALL, WHAT IS A CHAFFLE?

These "Chaffles" are nothing more than waffles made with cheese. Hence the name "Chaffle" which derives from the union "Cheese" + "Waf- fle". People tied to the keto diet usually love chaffles.

Grated cheese is a main ingredient in chaffle.

It's made with an egg and cheese batter instead of the flour-based batter you'll find in waffles. The high flour content in waffles adds a lot of carbohydrates, making them unhealthy according to the recommendations of the keto diet. Chaffles, on the other hand, have no flour. You can tell they're low-carb waffles with cheese.

The chaffles are extremely delicious. You won't realize that what you are actually eating is cheese eggs or cheese waffles. There are hundreds of chaffle recipes available, so you'll never miss out on options when you want to make one. There are also chaffles without cheese, for those who want to avoid or limit their intake of grated cheese.

CHAPTER 2

BENEFITS OF KETO DIET

The Keto diet has become so popular in recent years because of the success people have noticed. Not only have they lost weight, but scientific studies show that the Keto diet can help you improve your health in many others. As when starting any new diet or exercise routine, there may seem to be some disadvantages, so we will go over those for the Keto diet. But most people agree that the benefits outweigh the change period!

Benefits/Advantages

Losing weight: for most people, this is the foremost benefit of switching to Keto! Their previous diet method may have stalled for them, or they were noticing weight creeping back on. With Keto, studies have shown that people have been able to follow this diet and relay fewer hunger pangs and suppressed appetite while losing weight at the same time! You are minimizing your carbohydrate intake, which means more occasional blood sugar spikes. Often, those fluctuations in blood sugar levels make you feel hungrier and more prone to snacking in between meals. Instead, by guiding the body towards ketosis, you are eating a more fulfilling diet of fat and protein and harnessing energy from ketone molecules instead of glucose. Studies show that low-carb diets effectively reduce visceral fat (the fat you commonly see around the abdomen increases as you become obese). This reduces your risk of obesity and improves your health in the long run.

Reduce the Risk of Type 2 Diabetes:

The problem with carbohydrates is how unstable they make blood sugar levels. This can be very dangerous for people who have diabetes or are pre-diabetic because of unbalanced blood sugar levels or family history. Keto is an excellent option because of the minimal intake of carbohydrates it requires. Instead, you are harnessing most of your calories from fat or protein, which will not cause blood sugar spikes and, ultimately, less pressured the pancreas to secrete insulin. Many studies have found that diabetes patients who followed the Keto diet lost more weight and eventually reduced their fasting glucose levels. This is monumental news for patients with unstable blood sugar levels or hopes to avoid or reduce their diabetes medication intake.

Improve cardiovascular risk symptoms to lower your chances of having heart disease:

Most people assume that following Keto is so high in fat content has to increase your risk of coronary heart disease or heart attack. But the research proves otherwise! Research shows that switching to Keto can lower your blood pressure, increase your HDL good cholesterol, and reduce your triglyceride fatty acid levels. That's because the fat you are consuming on Keto is healthy and high-quality fats, so they reverse many unhealthy symptoms of heart disease. They boost your "good" HDL cholesterol numbers and decrease your "bad" LDL cholesterol numbers. It also reduces the level of triglyceride fatty acids in the bloodstream. A top-level of these can lead to stroke, heart attack, or prema- ture death. And what are the top levels of fatty acids linked to?

High Consumption of Carbohydrates:

With the Keto diet, you are drastically cutting your intake of carbohydrates to improve fatty acid levels and improve other risk factors. A 2018 study on the Keto diet found that it can improve 22 out of 26 risk factors for cardiovascular heart disease! These factors can be critical to some people, especially those who have a history of heart disease in their family.

Increases the Body's Energy Levels:

Let's briefly compare the difference between the glucose molecules synthesized from a high carbohydrate intake versus ketones produced on the Keto diet. The liver makes ketones and use fat molecules you already stored.

This makes themmuch more energy-rich and an endless source of fuel compared to glucose, a simple sugar molecule. These ketones

can give you a burst of energy physically and mentally, allowing you to have greater focus, clarity, and attention to detail.

Decreases inflammation in the body:

Inflammation on its own is a natural response by the body's immune system, but when it becomes uncontrollable, it can lead to an array of health problems, some severe and some minor. The health concerns include acne, autoimmune conditions, arthritis, psoriasis, irritable bowel syndrome, and even acne and eczema. Often, removing sugars and carbohydrates from your diet can help patients of these diseases avoid flare-ups - and the delightful news is Keto does just that! A 2008 research study found that Keto decreased a blood marker linked to high inflammation in the body by nearly 40%. This is glorious news for people who may suffer from inflammatory disease and want to change their diet to improve.

Increases your mental Functioning Level:

As we elaborated earlier, the energy-rich ketones can boost

the body's physical and mental levels of alertness. Research has shown that Keto is a much better energy source for the brain than simple sugar glucose molecules are. With nearly 75% of your diet coming from healthy fats, the brain's neural cells and mitochondria have a better source of energy to function at the highest level. Some studies have tested patients on the Keto diet and found they had higher cognitive functioning, better memory recall, and were less susceptible to memory loss. The Keto diet can even decrease the occurrence of migraines, which can be very detrimental to patients.

Decreases risk of diseases like Alzheimer's, Parkinson's, and epilepsy.

They created the Keto diet in the 1920s to combat epilepsy in children. From there, research has found that Keto can improve your cognitive functioning level and protect brain cells from injury or damage. This is very good to reduce the risk of neurodegenerative disease, which begins in the brain because of neural cells mutating and functioning with damaged parts or lower than peak optimal functioning.

Studies have found that the following Keto can improve the mental functioning of patients who suffer from diseases like Alzheimer's or Parkinson's. These neurodegenerative diseases sadly, have no cure, but the Keto diet could improve symptoms as they progress. Researchers believe that it's because of cutting out carbs from your diet, which reduces the occurrence of blood sugar spikes that the body's neural cells have to keep adjusting to.

Keto can regulate hormones in women who have PCOS (polycystic ovary syndrome) and PMS (pre-menstrual syndrome).

Women who have PCOS suffer from infertility, which can be very heartbreaking for young couples trying to start a family. For this condition, there is no known cure, but we believe it's related to many similar diabetic symptoms like obesity and a high level of insulin. This causes the body to produce more sex hormones, which can lead to infertility. The Keto diet paved its way as a popular way to regulate insulin and hormone levels and increase a woman's chances of getting pregnant.

Disadvantages

Your body will have a Changed period: It depends from person to person on the number of days that will be, but when you start any new diet or exercise routine, your body has to adjust to the new normal. With the Keto diet, you are drastically cutting your carbohydrates intake, so the body must adjust to that. You may feel slow, weak, exhausted, and like you are not thinking as quick or fast as you used to. It just means that your body is adjusting Keto, and once this change period is done, you will see the weight loss results you expected.

If you are an athlete, you may need more carbohydrates:

If you still want to try Keto as an athlete, you must talk to your nutritionist or trainer to see how the diet can be tweaked for you. Most athletes require a greater intake of carbs than the Keto diet requires, which means they may have to up their intake to ensure they have the energy for their training sessions. High endurance sports (like rugby or soccer) and

heavy weightlifting requires more significant information on carbohy- drates. If you're an athlete wanting to follow Keto and gain the health benefits, it's crucial you first talk to your trainer before changing your diet.

You have to count your daily macros carefully:

For beginners, this can be tough, and even people already on Keto can become lazy about this. People are often used to eating what they want without worrying about just how many grams of protein or carbs it contains. With Keto, be meticulous about counting your intake to ensure you are maintaining the Keto breakdown (75% fat, 20% protein, ~5% carbs). The closer you stick to this, the better results you will see regard- ing weight loss and other health benefits. If your weight loss has stalled or you're not feeling as energetic as you hoped, it could be because your macros are off. Find a free calorie counting app that you look at the ingredients of everything you're eating and cooking.

CHAPTER 3

HOW TO MAKE THE PERFECT CHAFFLE

Here are some tips that will help you make fantastic chaffles

•   Add a slice of chopped ham while mixing the egg and cheese. This will give you more protein and flavor. Those on a strict keto diet can also use bacon.

•   Before adding the egg and cheese mixture, sprinkle some extra cheese on your waffle or chaffle maker. You will then have a savory and crispy chaffle.

•   Don't open the waffle iron too early for checking. It should continue cooking until the chaffle is done and crisp. Let it cook for slightly longer for best results.

•   Use mozzarella if you want your chaffle to be sweet. Cheddar cheese is good for savory chaffles. You can use Haloumi or goat cheese, but mozzarella is always the best option because it is mild and not as greasy as many other cheese varieties. Mozzarella will also reduce the eggy taste.

•   Pepper jack cheese will give a slightly spicy taste. Almond/Coconut Flour in Chaffles

Chapter 4

SIMPLE CHAFFLE RECIPES

Chaffle bagels

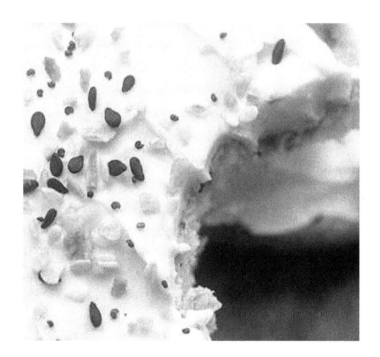

Servings: 2

Preparation time: 5 minutes Nutritional Values:

322 kcal Calories | 23 g Fat | 5 g Carbs | 19 g Proteins

Ingredients

- 1 large egg

- 1 tsp of coconut flour
- 1 tsp of everything bagel seasoning (and as well as more, for serving)
- 1/2 cup of mozzarella cheese, finely shredded
- 2 tbsp of cream cheese

Directions

Turn on to preheat your waffle iron

Stir the coconut flour, egg as well as bagel seasoning together till fully mixed. Mix the cheese in

Pour half the mixture of the eggs in the waffle iron then cook for about

3 min

Put the waffle out and continue with the egg mixture leftover

Layer each waffle of cream cheese then, if needed, sprinkle with extra bagel seasoning

Notes

To cut off a whole, from the waffle middle, use a sharp knife and make it look very much like a bagel, or just enjoy it like it is

Chaffles With Keto Ice Cream

Servings: 2

Cooking Time: 14 Minutes

Ingredients:

- 1 egg, beaten
- ½ cup finely grated mozzarella cheese
- ¼ cup almond flour
- 2 tbsp swerve confectioner's sugar
- 1/8 tsp xanthan gum
- Low-carb ice cream (flavor of your choice) for serving

Directions:

Preheat the waffle iron.

In a medium bowl, mix all the ingredients except the ice cream.

Open the iron and add half of the mixture. Close and cook until crispy, 7 minutes.

Transfer the chaffle to a plate and make second one with the remaining batter.

On each chaffle, add a scoop of low carb ice cream, fold into half-moons and enjoy.

Nutrition Info:

Calories 89;

Fats 48g; Carbs 1.67g; Net Carbs 1.37g; Protein 5.91g

Layered Cheese Chaffles

Servings: 1

Cooking Time: 5 Minutes

Ingredients:

- 1 organic egg, beaten
- 1/3 cup Cheddar cheese, shredded
- ½ teaspoon ground flaxseed
- ¼ teaspoon organic baking powder
- 2 tablespoons Parmesan cheese, shredded

Directions:

Preheat a mini waffle iron and then grease it.

In a bowl, place all the ingredients except Parmesan and beat until well combined.

Place half the Parmesan cheese in the bottom of preheated waffle iron. Place half of the egg mixture over cheese and top with the remaining Parmesan cheese.

Cook for about 3-minutes or until golden brown. Serve warm.

Nutrition Info:

Per Servings: Calories: 264

Net Carb: 1; Fat: 20g; Saturated Fat: 11.1g;

Carbohydrates: 2.1g; Dietary Fiber: 0.4g;

Sugar: 0.6g; Protein: 18.9g

Cajun, shrimp and avocado chaffle sandwich

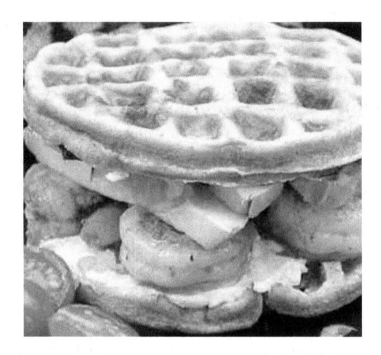

Servings: 2

Preparation time: 15 minutes Nutritional Values:

488 kcal Calories | 32.22 g Fat | 6.01g Carbs | 47.59g Proteins

Ingredients

Cajun aromatized chaffle

- 4 eggs, should be large
- 2 cups shredded mozzarella part-skim cheese
- 1 tsp Seasoning of Cajun Filling for sandwich
- 1-pound fresh shrimp peeled and deveined
- 1 tbsp of bacon (or avocado) grease
- 4 slices of bacon cooked

- 1 large sliced avocado
- 1/4 cup red onion, thinly sliced
- 1 dish bacon scallion cream cheese spread optional
- 1 Tsp Seasoning (Cajun)

Directions

Whisk the eggs together. Add 2 cups of mozzarella cheese with low moisture, and 1 tsp of Cajun seasoning. Put 1/4 cup of cheese and mix- ture of eggs over a mini waffle pan. Cook until the chaffle is browned. Repeat the process with the left egg and cheese batter

Add shrimp and combine it in a large bowl, with the remaining 1 tsp of Cajun seasoning. Garnish with salt and pepper. Fried in a pan over me- dium-high heat with bacon grease until the shrimp is translucent. Lift the fried shrimp and put aside. Let cool if desired

Place bacon scallion cream cheese over a side of a chaffle to create the Chaffle Sandwich: cover the top of the chaffle with shrimp, bacon, av- ocado and red onion. Cover with one more chaffle.

Serve as you wish

Vanilla Mozzarella Chaffles

Servings: 2

Cooking Time: 12 Minutes

Ingredients:

- 1 organic egg, beaten
- 1 teaspoon organic vanilla extract
- 1 tablespoon almond flour
- 1 teaspoon organic baking powder
- Pinch of ground cinnamon
- 1 cup Mozzarella cheese, shredded

Directions:

Preheat a mini waffle iron and then grease it.

In a bowl, place the egg and vanilla extract and beat until well combined. Add the flour, baking powder and cinnamon and mix well.

Add the Mozzarella cheese and stir to combine.

In a small bowl, place the egg and Mozzarella cheese and stir to combine. Place half of the mixture into preheated waffle iron and cook for about 5-minutes or until golden brown. Repeat with the remaining mixture. Serve warm.

Nutrition Info:

Per Servings: Calories: 103; Net Carb: 2.4g; Fat: 6.6g

Saturated Fat: 2.3g; Carbohydrates: 2; Dietary Fiber: 0.5g; Sugar: 0.6g; Protein: 6.8g

Bruschetta Chaffle

Servings: 2

Cooking Time: 5 Minutes

Ingredients:

- 2 basic chaffles
- 2 tablespoons sugar-free marinara sauce
- 2 tablespoons mozzarella, shredded
- 1 tablespoon olives, sliced
- 1 tomato sliced
- 1 tablespoon keto friendly pesto sauce
- Basil leaves

Directions:

Spread marinara sauce on each chaffle.

Spoon pesto and spread on top of the marinara sauce. Top with the tomato, olives and mozzarella.

Bake in the oven for 3 minutes or until the cheese has melted.

Garnish with basil.

Serve and enjoy.

Nutrition Info:

Calories 182; Total Fat 11g; Saturated Fat 6.1g;

Cholesterol 30mg; Sodium 508mg; Potassium 1mg;

Total Carbohydrate 3.1g; Dietary Fiber 1.1g; Protein 16.8g

Total Sugars 1g

Egg-free Psyllium Husk Chaffles

Servings: 1

Cooking Time: 4 Minutes

Ingredients:

- 1-ounce Mozzarella cheese, shredded
- 1 tablespoon cream cheese, softened
- 1 tablespoon psyllium husk powder

Directions:

Preheat a waffle iron and then grease it.

In a blender, place all ingredients and pulse until a slightly crumbly mix- ture forms.

Place the mixture into preheated waffle iron and cook for about 4 min- utes or until golden brown.

Serve warm.

Nutrition Info:

Per Servings:

Calories: 137 Net Carb: 1.3g Fat: 8.8g Saturated Fat: 2g Carbohydrates: 1.3g Dietary Fiber: 0g Sugar: 0g Protein: 9.5g

Mozzarella & Almond Flour Chaffles

Servings: 2

Cooking Time: 8 Minutes

Ingredients:

- ½ cup Mozzarella cheese, shredded
- 1 large organic egg
- 2 tablespoons blanched almond flour
- ¼ teaspoon organic baking powder

Directions:

Preheat a mini waffle iron and then grease it.

In a medium bowl, place all ingredients and with a fork, mix until well combined.

Place half of the mixture into preheated waffle iron and cook for about 4 minutes or until golden brown.

Repeat with the remaining mixture. Serve warm.

Nutrition Info:

Per Servings: Calories: 98 Net Carb: 1.4g Fat: 7.1g Saturated Fat: 1g Carbohydrates: 2.2g Dietary Fiber: 0.8g Sugar: 0.2g Protein: 7g

Keto chocolate chaffle recipe

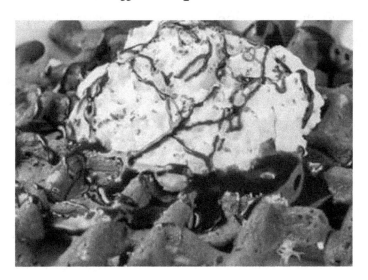

Servings: 1

Preparation Time: 10 min Nutritional Value:

672 kcal Calories | 70 g Fat | 11 g Carbs | 13 g Proteins

Ingredients

- 1/2 cup of sugar-free Choco-chips
- 1/2 cup of butter
- 3 eggs
- 1/4 cup of Truvia, or any other sweetener
- 1 tsp of vanilla extract

Directions

Melt the chocolate and butter in a secure bowl in the microwave for

around 1 min

Remove it and mix it excellently

You ought to just use the heat inside chocolate and butter to melt the remaining clumps. You've over-cooked the chocolate when your micro-wave till it's melted it all

Then have a spoon, as well as start to mix

If necessary, add 10 sec but mix just before you intend to do so Put the sweetener, vanilla and the eggs in a bowl and combine until it becomes light and foamy

In a gradual flow, add the melted chocolate and butter into the bowl, then beat it again till well absorbed

Place approximately 1/4 of the blend into a Mini Waffle Maker, then cook for 7-8 mins or till it becomes crispy

Should produce four waffles, leftover with just a little batter

Tips

- For higher results, serve this one with syrup or whipped cream when warm.
- Don't over-heat the chocolate; it will burn. Only cook and mix until soft & melted.

Pulled Pork Chaffle Sandwiches

Servings: 4

Cooking Time: 28 Minutes

Ingredients:

- 2 eggs, beaten
- 1 cup finely grated cheddar cheese
- ¼ tsp baking powder
- 2 cups cooked and shredded pork
- 1 tbsp sugar-free BBQ sauce
- 2 cups shredded coleslaw mix
- 2 tbsp apple cider vinegar
- ½ tsp salt
- ¼ cup ranch dressing

Directions:

Preheat the waffle iron.

In a medium bowl, mix the eggs, cheddar cheese, and baking powder. Open the iron and add a quarter of the mixture. Close and cook until crispy, 7 minutes.

Transfer the chaffle to a plate and make 3 more chaffles in the same manner.

Meanwhile, in another medium bowl, mix the pulled pork with the BBQ sauce until well combined. Set aside.

Also, mix the coleslaw mix, apple cider vinegar, salt, and ranch dressing in another medium bowl.

When the chaffles are ready, on two pieces, divide the pork and then top with the ranch coleslaw. Cover with the remaining chaffles and insert mini skewers to secure the sandwiches.

Enjoy afterward.

Nutrition Info:

Calories 374; Fats 23.61g; Carbs 8.2g; Net Carbs 8.2g; Protein 28.05g

Cheddar & Egg White Chaffles

Servings: 4

Cooking Time: 12 Minutes

Ingredients:

- 2 egg whites
- 1 cup Cheddar cheese, shredded

Directions:

Preheat a mini waffle iron and then grease it.

In a small bowl, place the egg whites and cheese and stir to combine. Place ¼ of the mixture into preheated waffle iron and cook for about 4 minutes or until golden brown.

Repeat with the remaining mixture. Serve warm.

Nutrition Info:

Per Servings: Calories: 122; Net Carb: 0.5g; Fat: 9.4g; Saturated Fat: Carbohydrates: 0.5g; Dietary Fiber: 0g Sugar: 0.3g; Protein: 8.8g

Creamy Chicken Chaffle Sandwich

Servings: 2

Cooking Time: 10 Minutes

Ingredients:

- Cooking spray
- 1 cup chicken breast fillet, cubed
- Salt and pepper to taste
- ¼ cup all-purpose cream
- 4 garlic chaffles
- Parsley, chopped

Directions:

Spray your pan with oil. Put it over medium heat.

Add the chicken fillet cubes. Season with salt and pepper. Reduce heat and add the cream.

Spread chicken mixture on top of the chaffle. Garnish with parsley and top with another chaffle.

Nutrition Info: Calories 273;

Total Fat 34g;

Saturated Fat 4.1g; Cholesterol 62mg; Sodium 373mg;

Total Carbohydrate 22.5g; Dietary Fiber 1.1g;

Total Sugars 3.2g; Protein 17.5g; Potassium 177mg

Spicy Shrimp and Chaffles

Servings: 4

Cooking Time: 31 Minutes

Ingredients:

- For the shrimp:
- 1 tbsp olive oil
- 1 lb jumbo shrimp, peeled and deveined
- 1 tbsp Creole seasoning
- Salt to taste
- 2 tbsp hot sauce
- 3 tbsp butter
- 2 tbsp chopped fresh scallions to garnish
- For the chaffles:
- 2 eggs, beaten
- 1 cup finely grated Monterey Jack cheese

Directions:

For the shrimp:

Heat the olive oil in a medium skillet over medium heat.

Season the shrimp with the Creole seasoning and salt. Cook in the oil until pink and opaque on both sides, 2 minutes.

Pour in the hot sauce and butter. Mix well until the shrimp is adequately coated in the sauce, 1 minute.

Turn the heat off and set aside. For the chaffles:

Preheat the waffle iron.

In a medium bowl, mix the eggs and Monterey Jack cheese.

Open the iron and add a quarter of the mixture. Close and cook until crispy, 7 minutes.

Transfer the chaffle to a plate and make 3 more chaffles in the same manner.

Cut the chaffles into quarters and place on a plate. Top with the shrimp and garnish with the scallions. Serve warm.

Nutrition Info:

Calories 342Fats; 19.75g; Carbs 2.8g; Net Carbs 2.3g; Protein 36.01g

Strawberry Shortcake Chaffle Bowls

Servings: 4

Cooking Time: 28 Minutes

Ingredients:

- 1 egg, beaten
- ½ cup finely grated mozzarella cheese
- 1 tbsp almond flour
- ¼ tsp baking powder
- 2 drops cake batter extract
- 1 cup cream cheese, softened
- 1 cup fresh strawberries, sliced
- 1 tbsp sugar-free maple syrup

Directions:

Preheat a waffle bowl maker and grease lightly with cooking spray. Meanwhile, in a medium bowl, whisk all the ingredients except the cream cheese and strawberries.

Open the iron, pour in half of the mixture, cover, and cook until crispy, 6 to 7 minutes.

Remove the chaffle bowl onto a plate and set aside. Make a second chaffle bowl with the remaining batter.

To serve, divide the cream cheese into the chaffle bowls and top with the strawberries.

Drizzle the filling with the maple syrup and serve.

Nutrition Info:

Calories 235; Fats 20.62g; Carbs 5.9g; Net Carbs 5g; Protein 7.51g

Pumpkin & Pecan Chaffle

Servings: 2

Cooking Time: 10 Minutes

Ingredients:

- 1 egg, beaten
- ½ cup mozzarella cheese, grated
- ½ teaspoon pumpkin spice
- 1 tablespoon pureed pumpkin
- 2 tablespoons almond flour
- 1 teaspoon sweetener
- 2 tablespoons pecans, chopped

Directions:

Turn on the waffle maker. Beat the egg in a bowl.

Stir in the rest of the ingredients.

Pour half of the mixture into the device. Seal the lid.

Cook for 5 minutes.

Remove the chaffle carefully.

Repeat the steps to make the second chaffle.

Nutrition Info: Calories 210;

Total Fat 17 g; Saturated Fat 10 g; Cholesterol 110 mg;

Sodium 250 mg; Potassium 570 mg;

Total Carbohydrate 4.6 g; Dietary Fiber 1.7 g;

Protein 11 g; Total Sugars 2 g

Chaffle Cannoli

Servings: 4

Cooking Time: 28 Minutes

Ingredients:

- For the chaffles:
- 1 large egg
- 1 egg yolk
- 3 tbsp butter, melted
- 1 tbso swerve confectioner's
- 1 cup finely grated Parmesan cheese
- 2 tbsp finely grated mozzarella cheese
- For the cannoli filling:
- ½ cup ricotta cheese
- 2 tbsp swerve confectioner's sugar
- 1 tsp vanilla extract
- 2 tbsp unsweetened chocolate chips for garnishing

Directions:

Preheat the waffle iron.

Meanwhile, in a medium bowl, mix all the ingredients for the chaffles. Open the iron, pour in a quarter of the mixture, cover, and cook until crispy, 7 minutes.

Remove the chaffle onto a plate and make 3 more with the remaining batter.

Meanwhile, for the cannoli filling:

Beat the ricotta cheese and swerve confectioner's sugar until smooth. Mix in the vanilla.

On each chaffle, spread some of the filling and wrap over. Garnish the creamy ends with some chocolate chips.

Serve immediately.

Nutrition Info:

Calories 308; Fats 25.05g; Carbs 5.17g; Net Carbs 5.17g; Protein 15.18g

Banananut Chaffle

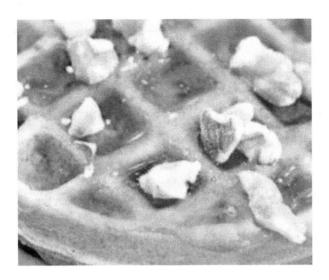

Servings: 2

Preparation time: 5 minutes Nutritional Values:

119 kcal Calories | 8 g Fats |

2.7 g Carbs | 9 g Proteins

Ingredients

- 1 egg
- 1 tbsp of cream cheese, soft plus at room temperature
- 1 tbsp of cheesecake pudding, sugar-free, optional
- 1/2 cup of mozzarella cheese
- 1 tbsp of Monk Fruit
- 1/4 tsp of vanilla extract
- 1/4 tsp of banana extract Toppings (optional)
- Caramel sauce, sugar-free
- Pecans

Directions

Heat up your waffle maker Whisk the egg in a little bowl

Transfer the rest of the ingredient to the mixture of the eggs, then com- bine until completely incorporated

Transfer half the mixture to the maker then cook till it is golden brown, for a duration of four minutes. Remove the cooked chaffle as well as put the other portion of the mixture to make the next chaffle

Top with the ingredients of your choice and serve hot

Keto Chaffle Sausage and Egg Breakfast Sandwich

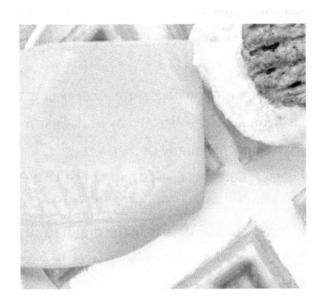

Servings: 2-3

Preparation time: 15 minutes Nutritional values:

433 kcal Calories | 28.4g Fat | 8.5g Carbs | 17.6g Proteins

Ingredients

- 2 large raw eggs
- 2 tbsp of coconut flour
- 2 tbsp mayo
- ½ tsp baking powder
- 1 tsp absolute substitute icing sugar by swerve
- 1 x 2 patties brown banquet, and serve patties
- 3 /4 ounces - 2 slice American cheese slices

Directions

At medium-high temperature, preheat the waffle iron. In a big mixing dish, add two whites, coconut flour, mayo, baking powder and whisk Whisk well. Let the batter stay for around 1 minute to thicken

Spray waffle iron with nonstick spray high heat grill. Put into hot waffle iron and cook as directed by iron. Take away waffles from the iron. Slice the chaffle in half

Meanwhile, use a nonstick cooking spray with a 4 oz ramekin. Add one egg and gently scramble it with a fork. Place completely cooked sausage patty in the middle and microwave for around 1 minute on 60 percent power before the egg is cooked through

Put egg and sausage with a slice of American cheese on a quarter of the chaffle. Repeat on the other sandwich with the cooking of another egg and sausage. Right away, enjoy or freeze in plastic wrap

Chocolate Melt Chaffles

Servings: 4

Cooking Time: 36 Minutes

Ingredients:

- For the chaffles:
- 2 eggs, beaten
- ¼ cup finely grated Gruyere cheese
- 2 tbsp heavy cream
- 1 tbsp coconut flour
- 2 tbsp cream cheese, softened
- 3 tbsp unsweetened cocoa powder
- 2 tsp vanilla extract
- A pinch of salt
- For the chocolate sauce:
- 1/3 cup + 1 tbsp heavy cream
- 1 ½ oz unsweetened baking chocolate, chopped
- 1 ½ tsp sugar-free maple syrup
- 1 ½ tsp vanilla extract

Directions:

For the chaffles:

Preheat the waffle iron.

In a medium bowl, mix all the ingredients for the chaffles.

Open the iron and add a quarter of the mixture. Close and cook until crispy, 7 minutes.

Transfer the chaffle to a plate and make 3 more with the remaining batter. For the chocolate sauce:

Pour the heavy cream into saucepan and simmer over low heat, 3 min- utes.

Turn the heat off and add the chocolate. Allow melting for a few minutes and stir until fully melted, 5 minutes.

Mix in the maple syrup and vanilla extract.

Assemble the chaffles in layers with the chocolate sauce sandwiched be- tween each layer.

Slice and serve immediately.

Nutrition Info:

Calories 172;

Fats 13.57g; Carbs 6.65g; Net Carbs 3.65g; Protein 5.76g

Low Carb Chaffle Bowl

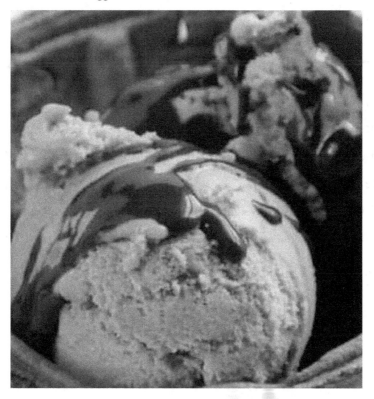

Servings: 1

Preparation time: 5 minutes Nutritional Values:

150 kcal Calories | 17g Fat | 3g Carbs | 7g Proteins

Ingredients

- 1 whipped egg
- 1 scoop of keto meal chocolate
- 1 tbsp of almond flour
- 1/4 tsp of baking powder

Directions

Preheat then sprinkle the "Bowl Waffle Maker" with non-stick cooking

oil

Break the egg in a little bowl. Whisk the egg

Add in the almond flour, keto meal and baking powder Mix till the components completely come together

Put the material around 1 minute to 1.5 minute into the heated waffle maker. When you see steam come out of the maker, you'll realize it's nearly done

Utilize tongs to consider removing the hot chaffle bowl from the maker

Let it cool down and enjoy it

Spicy Jalapeno & Bacon Chaffles

Servings:2

Cooking Time: 5 Minutes

Ingredients:

- 1 oz. cream cheese
- 1 large egg
- 1/2 cup cheddar cheese
- 2 tbsps. bacon bits
- 1/2 tbsp. jalapenos
- 1/4 tsp baking powder

Directions:

Switch on your waffle maker.

Grease your waffle maker with cooking spray and let it heat up. Mix together egg and vanilla extract in a bowl first.

Add baking powder, jalapenos and bacon bites. Add in cheese last and mix together.

Pour the chaffles batter intothe maker and cook the chaffles for about 2-3 minutesutes.

Once chaffles are cooked, remove from the maker.

Serve hot and enjoy!

Nutrition Info:

Per Servings: Protein: 24% 5kcal; Fat: 70% 175 kcal

Carbohydrates: 6% 15 kcal

Cheddar & Almond Flour Chaffles

Servings: 2

Cooking Time: 10 Minutes

Ingredients:

- 1 large organic egg, beaten
- ½ cup Cheddar cheese, shredded
- 2 tablespoons almond flour

Directions:

Preheat a mini waffle iron and then grease it.

In a bowl, place the egg, Cheddar cheese and almond flour and beat until well combined.

Place half of the mixture into preheated waffle iron and cook for about 5 minutes or until golden brown.

Repeat with the remaining mixture. Serve warm.

Nutrition Info:

Per Servings: Calories: 195; Net Carb: 1g; Fat: 15;

Saturated Fat: 7g; Carbohydrates: 1.8g; Dietary Fiber: 0.8g

Sugar: 0.6g; Protein: 10.2g

Keto Turkey Brie Cranberry Chaffle Sandwich

Servings: 1

Preparation time: 5 minutes Nutritional values:

537 kcal Calories | 36 g Fat |

8.6 g Carbs | 44 g Proteins

Ingredients

- 1/2 cup grated mozzarella
- 1 medium beaten egg
- 2 tbsp of almond flour Filling
- 2 slices of turkey
- 3 Slices Brie
- 2 tbsp chia cranberry jam

Directions

Turn your waffle maker on and grease it gently

Add the egg, mozzarella, and almond flour in a bowl. Combine until mixed

Spoon the mixture into the waffle maker. If you want a small waffle mak- er, spoon half the batter in at a time)

Close the lid and cook until golden and firm for 5 minutes Use tongs to remove the cooked waffles and set aside

Place the turkey, brie, and cranberry on a cutting board and layer on chaffle. Put the layers together with your choice

Place on top of the other chaffle and sliced in half

If you just want a warm sandwich, then heat it up for 20 seconds in the microwave

Simple& Beginner Chaffle

Servings:2

Cooking Time: 5 Minutes

Ingredients:

- 1 large egg
- 1/2 cup mozzarella cheese, shredded
- Cooking spray

Directions:

Switch on your waffle maker.

Beat the egg with a fork in a small mixing bowl.

Once the egg is beaten, add the mozzarella and mix well. Spray the waffle makerwith cooking spray.

Pour the chaffles mixture in a preheated waffle maker and let it cook for about 2-3 minutes.

Once the chaffles are cooked, carefully remove them from the maker and cook the remaining batter.

Serve hot with coffee and enjoy!

Nutrition Info:

Per Servings:

Protein: 36% 42 kcal; Fat 60% 71 kcal;

Carbohydrates: 4% 5 kcal

Arby's Chaffle

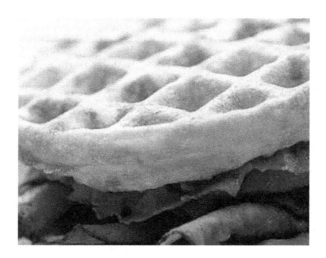

Servings: 2-3

Preparation time: 15 minutes Nutritional Values:

386 kcal Calories | 20 g Fat | 8 g Carbs | 40 g Proteins

Ingredients

For beef:

- 1/2 cup of beef broth
- 4 oz of deli roast beef, thinly sliced for chaffle bun:
- 1 beaten egg
- 1 tsp of coconut flour
- 1/4 tsp of baking powder
- 1/2 cup of mozzarella, finely sliced Arby's sauce-low carb:
- 1 tbsp of ketchup, sugar-free
- 2 tsp of salad dressing, Italian
- 1/4 tsp of Worcestershire sauce
- 1/4 tsp of chopped pepper

Directions

For beef:

Add the broth of beef to a pan and take it to a boiling point. Include the beef in it and cook over low to warm the beef for five min. Cover it D and put aside when the chaffle is being prepared

For chaffle:

Switch on to preheat your waffle maker

Mix the coconut flour, egg as well as baking powder together. Then add the mozzarella in, and mix

In waffle iron, pour half of the mixture. Lock the waffle machine and cook for three minutes. Take the waffle out and proceed with batter left over

For Arby's sauce:

Mix all ingredients together to make the Arby's sauce To assemble:

Put the beef on one of the chaffles as well as drizzle it with Arby's sauce. Put the second chaffle over it

Eat immediately Notes

•When preparing an onion bun, scatter over the chaffles the finely chopped dried onion.

•If you are an Arby sauce eater, you will need to double the recipe of

sauce!

Keto Wonder-Bread Chaffle Sandwich

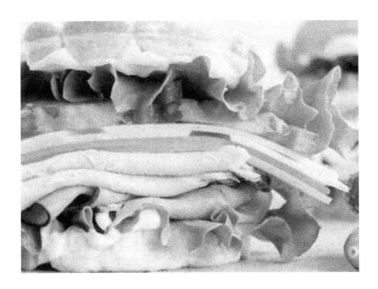

Serving: 2

Preparation time: 10 minutes Nutritional values:

208 kcal Calories | 17.4g Fat | 2.1g Carbs | 10.3g Proteins

Ingredients for wonder-bread chaffle

- 2 eggs white
- 2 tbsp of almond flour
- 1 tbsp mayonnaise
- 1 tsp of water
- 1/4 tsp baking powder
- 1 pinch salt

Ingredients for sandwich elements

- 2 tbsp mayonnaise
- 1-piece deli ham
- 1 slice deli turkey

- 1 slice of cheese cheddar
- 1 tomato slice
- 1 leaf green leaf lettuce

Directions

Preheat the maker. Mix all the ingredients of the wonder-bread chaffle in a tiny bowl. White bread chaffle components combined together in a large bowl

Place 1/2 the batter into the waffle maker and cook for about 3 to 5 min- utes until finished

Wonder-bread chaffle batter in a little waffle-maker

Remove the waffle when cooking has been completed. Repeat for the batter remaining

Made keto sandwich bread in a waffle maker

Place mayonnaise on one side of each bread chaffle sandwich. Place in green leaf, tomato and cold cuts

Asian Cauliflower Chaffles

Servings: 4

Cooking Time: 28 Minutes

Ingredients:

- For the chaffles:
- 1 cup cauliflower rice, steamed
- 1 large egg, beaten
- Salt and freshly ground black pepper to taste
- 1 cup finely grated Parmesan cheese
- 1 tsp sesame seeds
- ¼ cup chopped fresh scallions
- For the dipping sauce:
- 3 tbsp coconut aminos
- 1 ½ tbsp plain vinegar
- 1 tsp fresh ginger puree
- 1 tsp fresh garlic paste
- 3 tbsp sesame oil
- 1 tsp fish sauce
- 1 tsp red chili flakes

Directions:

Preheat the waffle iron.

In a medium bowl, mix the cauliflower rice, egg, salt, black pepper, and Parmesan cheese.

Open the iron and add a quarter of the mixture. Close and cook until crispy, 7 minutes.

Transfer the chaffle to a plate and make 3 more chaffles in the same manner.

Meanwhile, make the dipping sauce.

In a medium bowl, mix all the ingredients for the dipping sauce.

Plate the chaffles, garnish with the sesame seeds and scallions and serve with the dipping sauce.

Nutrition Info:

Calories 231; Fats 188g; Carbs 6.32g; Net Carbs 5.42g; Protein 9.66g

Egg-free Almond Flour Chaffles

Servings: 2

Cooking Time: 10 Minutes

Ingredients:

- 2 tablespoons cream cheese, softened
- 1 cup mozzarella cheese, shredded
- 2 tablespoons almond flour
- 1 teaspoon organic baking powder

Directions:

Preheat a mini waffle iron and then grease it.

In a medium bowl, place all ingredients and with a fork, mix until well combined.

Place half of the mixture into preheated waffle iron and cook for about 4-5 minutes or until golden brown.

Repeat with the remaining mixture. Serve warm.

Nutrition Info:

Per Servings: Calories: 77; Net Carb: 2.4g; Fat: 9.8g; Saturated Fat: 4g; Carbohydrates: 3.2g; Dietary Fiber: 0.8g; Sugar: 0.3g; Protein: 4.8g

Keto Chocolate Fudge Chaffle

Servings: 2

Cooking Time: 14 Minutes

Ingredients:

- 1 egg, beaten
- ¼ cup finely grated Gruyere cheese
- 2 tbsp unsweetened cocoa powder
- ¼ tsp baking powder
- ¼ tsp vanilla extract
- 2 tbsp erythritol
- 1 tsp almond flour
- 1 tsp heavy whipping cream
- A pinch of salt

Directions:

Preheat the waffle iron.

Add all the ingredients to a medium bowl and mix well.

Open the iron and add half of the mixture. Close and cook until golden brown and crispy, 7 minutes.

Remove the chaffle onto a plate and make another with the remaining batter.

Cut each chaffle into wedges and serve after.

Nutrition Info: Per Servings: Calories 173; Fats 13.08g; Carbs 3.98g; Net Carbs 2.28g; Protein 12.27g

Keto Chaffle Cuban Sandwich

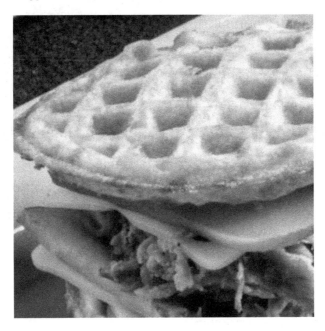

Servings: 1-2

Preparation time: 10 minutes Nutritional values:

522 kcal Calories | 33 g Fat | 4 g Carbs | 46 g Proteins

Ingredients

- 1 large egg
- 1 tbsp of almond flour
- 1 tbsp of Greek full fat yogurt
- 1/8 tsp baking powder
- 1/4 cup swiss cheese crushed

For filling the sandwich

- 3 ounces roast pork
- 2 once deli ham
- 1 slice of Swiss cheese

- Chips of 3 to 5 pickles, sliced
- 1/2 tbsp Dijon mustard

Directions

Preheat your waffle iron

In a small bowl, mix the egg, yogurt, almond flour and baking powder together

Scatter one fourth of the Swiss shredded straight onto the hot waffle iron. Cover with half of the mixture of egg, then apply 1/4 more Swiss on it. Cover the iron and cook until light brown and crunchy for 3-5 minutes Repeat the same procedure with the ingredients left behind

For the fillings in sandwich

In a small microwaveable dish, place the pork, Swiss cheese slice and ham in order. Microwave the cheese for 40 to 50 sec, before it melts Cover with the mustard on the inner part of one chaffle, then finish with pickles. Reverse the bowl, so the molten Swiss hits the pickles on top of the chaffle. Put the chaffle at bottom on the roast pork & reverse the sandwich to keep the side of pork below and the side of mustard up

Keto Reuben Sandwich Chaffle

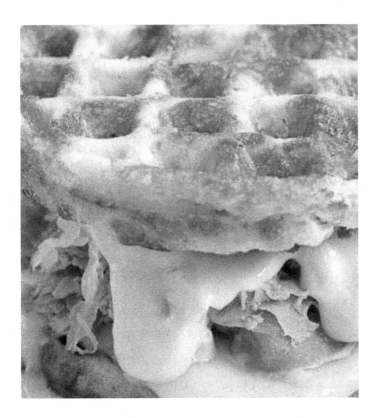

Servings: 1

Preparation time: 6 minutes Nutritional values:

605 kcal Calories | 43.8 g Fat |

6.8 g Carbs | 45.1 g Proteins

Ingredients

- 1 egg
- 1/2 cup mozzarella cheese
- 2 tbsp of flour (almond)
- 2 tbsp of low carbohydrate thousand island dressing

- 1/4 tsp baking powder
- 1/4 tsp of seeds of caraway
- 2 corned beef slices
- 1 Swiss cheese slice
- 2 tbsp of sauerkraut

Directions

set the temperature to the mid-high heat of the waffle maker

In a bowl, mix together the egg, mozzarella, almond flour, a tbsp of low carb dressing seeds of caraway as well as baking powder

Place the chaffle batter into the waffle maker center. Shut the waffle ma- chine and let it be cooked for 5 to 7 min or till lightly browned and crisp is perfect. If a mini waffle maker is used, just spill half the mixture over the waffle machine. Two chaffles (mini) will be produced from this recipe Take chaffle out from the waffle machine. If you are using a mini waffle machine, repeat for the residual batter

Place the corned beef on a sheet of parchment, and cover with a Swiss cheese slice. Heat for 20 to 30 sec in the oven, before the cheese begins to melt. Take off from the microwave. Place on each chaffle the remain- ing tbsp of low carbohydrate thousand island sauce spread the Swiss cheese and hot corned beef, and finish with sauerkraut as well as other chaffle

Broccoli & Cheese Chaffle

Servings: 2

Cooking Time: 8 Minutes

Ingredients:

- ¼ cup broccoli florets
- 1 egg, beaten
- 1 tablespoon almond flour
- ¼ teaspoon garlic powder
- ½ cup cheddar cheese

Directions:

Preheat your waffle maker.

Add the broccoli to the food processor. Pulse until chopped. Add to a bowl.

Stir in the egg and the rest of the ingredients. Mix well.

Pour half of the batter to the waffle maker. Cover and cook for 4 minutes.

Repeat procedure to make the next chaffle.

Nutrition Info:

Calories 170;

Total Fat 13 g; Saturated Fat 7 g; Cholesterol 112 mg;

Sodium 211 mg; Potassium 94 mg; Total Carbohydrate 2 g;

Dietary Fiber 1 g; Protein 11 g; Total Sugars 1 g

Zucchini Parmesan Chaffles

Servings: 2

Cooking Time: 14 Minutes

Ingredients:

- 1 cup shredded zucchini
- 1 egg, beaten
- ½ cup finely grated Parmesan cheese
- Salt and freshly ground black pepper to taste

Directions:

Preheat the waffle iron.

Put all the ingredients in a medium bowl and mix well.

Open the iron and add half of the mixture. Close and cook until crispy, 7 minutes.

Remove the chaffle onto a plate and make another with the remaining mixture.

Cut each chaffle into wedges and serve afterward.

Nutrition Info:

Per Servings: Calories 138; Fats 9.07g; Carbs 3.81g; Net Carbs 3.71g; Protein 10.02g

Cream Cheese Chaffle With Lemon Curd

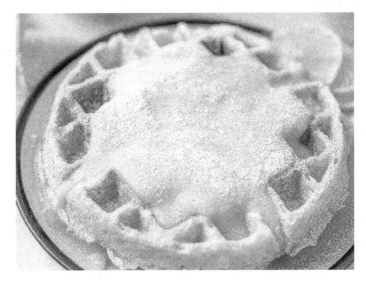

Servings: 2

Preparation Time: 5 min Nutritional Values:

302 kcal Calories | 24 g Fat | 6 g Carbs | 15 g Proteins

Ingredients

- 1 batch keto lemon curd
- 3 large eggs
- 4 oz of softened cream cheese
- 1 tbsp of low carbohydrate sweetener
- 1 tsp of vanilla extract
- 3/4 cup of shredded mozzarella cheese
- 3 tbsp of coconut flour
- 1 tsp of baking powder
- 1/3 tsp of salt
- keto whipped cream, homemade (additional and optional)

Directions

Make lemon curd, and then let chill in the fridge

In the meantime, warm up your waffle maker and oil it like you usually do

Put baking powder, coconut flour and salt in a little bowl. Mix together

and put away

Put the eggs, sweetener, vanilla and cream cheese into a large bowl. Beat till frothy by using a hand beater. You might have blocks of remaining cream cheese, so that's okay

Combine the egg mixture with the mozzarella cheese and keep beating Put dry ingredients into the mixture and proceed to mix until well mixed Put batter in the hot waffle maker and prepare a waffle as you do. Some- times a few mins

Take away from waffle processor, coat with cooled lemon curd, then serve with optional whipped cream

Keto French Dip Chaffwich

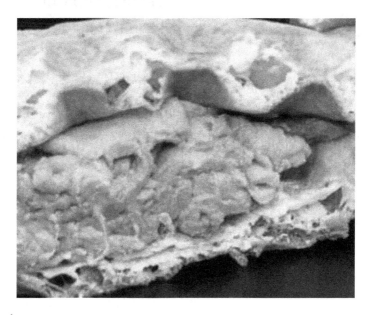

Servings: 1-2

Preparation time: 10 minutes Nutritional values:

444 kcal Calories | 26 g Fat | 6 g Carbs | 45 g Proteins

Ingredients

- 4 ounces of roasted beef
- 2 eggs (egg whites only)
- 2 tbsp almond flour
- 1 tbsp of sour cream
- 1-1/2 cup mozzarella
- 1/2 cup beef broth low in sodium

Directions

Whip the egg white till foamy, to make the chaffle. Include the almond flour and sour cream and mix properly. Add the cheese in

Heat up the mini waffle maker according to instructions from the manufacturer. Add half the batter when heated and cook for 7-10 mins once the chaffle is nicely browned and readily releases. Repeat with the batter left behind

In the meanwhile, heat the beef broth in a tiny pot or pan. Heat up the sliced beef, don't overcook it!

Put the processed beef on the chaffle to be assembled, top with cheese and serve sideways with the available broth

Keto Ham and Cheese Chaffle Sandwich

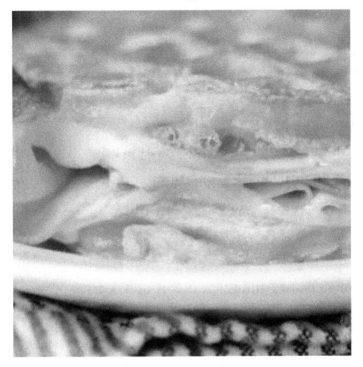

Servings: 1

Preparation Time: 15 Minutes Nutritional Values:

733 Kcal Calories | 57.1g Fat | 8.4g Carbs | 45.8g Proteins

Ingredients

- 1 egg, should be large
- 1/2 cup crushed cheddar, mozzarella or any grated cheese
- 1/4 cup almond flour.
- 1/4 tsp gluten-free baking powder
- 2 ham slices
- 57g - 2 slices of cheese

- 4 - 60g tomato slices
- 15g - 2 small leaves of lettuce
- Optional: 1 or 2 tbsp of cream cheese, butter, or mayonnaise.

Directions

Start making the chaffles as per the directions. Either you can create 2 standard chaffles, or 3 thinner ones

Let the chaffles all cool down. They will be soft when hot but will crisp when getting colder

Fill with ham, cheese, lettuce and tomato croutons. Optionally, before filling, you can add 1 to 2 spoonsful of cream cheese and spread it over the chaffles

Immediately enjoy or place the chaffles in a sealed container for up to 3 days at room temperature or in the refrigerator for up to a week. Freeze for up to 3 months, for longer storage. The jar would maintain the soft texture, but if you want crispy, you should leave them untouched

Fudgy Chocolate Desert Chaffles

Servings: 4

Preparation time: 5 minutes Nutritional Values:

83 kcal Calories | 5.4 g Fat | 3 g Carbs | 6.1 g Proteins

Ingredients

- 2 eggs, large
- 2 tbsp whipping cream, heavy
- 4 tbsp of crushed mozzarella cheese
- 1 tbsp of dark cacao
- 2 tsp of coconut flour
- 1/2 tsp of baking powder (gluten-free)
- 1/2 tsp of vanilla extract (gluten-free)
- 1/4 tsp of stevia powder
- A pinch of salt

Directions

Get your waffle maker preheated. Sprinkle gently with cooking spray (high-heat)

Whip the eggs as well as cream in a bowl. Insert the rest of the ingredients, then mix to blend

When you have heated the waffle iron, spread the mixture in the fillable parts, making sure not to overload the area of the plate

Shut the cover to cook. There might be some steam coming from the edges as the chaffles cook, and the cover will rise gradually as they cook Both are indications that tasty chaffles are on the way

Cook them for 3 to 5 min till the indicator light is turned green, or when the upper cover moves easily as well as the chaffles appear fluffy and brownish. Carefully remove the chaffles from the waffle maker, because it is really hot

Repeat 3 & 4 steps until the residual batter is used

Put in the plate, then serve as a low-carb snack with whipped cream & fruit, or (sugar-free) ice cream

Chaffled Brownie Sundae

Servings: 4

Cooking Time: 30 Minutes

Ingredients:

- For the chaffles:
- 2 eggs, beaten
- 1 tbsp unsweetened cocoa powder
- 1 tbsp erythritol
- 1 cup finely grated mozzarella cheese
- For the topping:
- 3 tbsp unsweetened chocolate, chopped
- 3 tbsp unsalted butter
- ½ cup swerve sugar
- Low-carb ice cream for topping
- 1 cup whipped cream for topping
- 3 tbsp sugar-free caramel sauce

Directions:

For the chaffles:

Preheat the waffle iron.

Meanwhile, in a medium bowl, mix all the ingredients for the chaffles. Open the iron, pour in a quarter of the mixture, cover, and cook until crispy, 7 minutes.

Remove the chaffle onto a plate and make 3 more with the remaining batter.

Plate and set aside. For the topping:

Meanwhile, melt the chocolate and butter in a medium saucepan with occasional stirring, 2 minutes.

To Servings:

Divide the chaffles into wedges and top with the ice cream, whipped cream, and swirl the chocolate sauce and caramel sauce on top.

Serve immediately.

Nutrition Info: Calories 165 | Fats 11.39g | Carbs 3.81g | Net Carbs 2.91g | Protein 79g

Keto Chaffle Sandwich Recipes

Chicken Jalapeño Chaffles

Servings: 2

Cooking Time: 14 Minutes

Ingredients:

- 1/8 cup finely grated Parmesan cheese
- ¼ cup finely grated cheddar cheese
- 1 egg, beaten
- ½ cup cooked chicken breasts, diced
- 1 small jalapeño pepper, deseeded and minced
- 1/8 tsp garlic powder
- 1/8 tsp onion powder
- 1 tsp cream cheese, softened

Directions:

Preheat the waffle iron.

In a medium bowl, mix all the ingredients until adequately combined. Open the iron and add half of the mixture. Close and cook until crispy, 7 minutes.

Transfer the chaffle to a plate and make a second chaffle in the same manner.

Allow cooling and serve afterward.

Nutrition Info:

Calories 201 | Fats 11.49g | Carbs 3.7 | Net Carbs 3.36g | Protein 20.11g

Keto Red Velvet Chaffle Cake

Servings: 1

Preparation Time: 20 Minutes Nutritional Values:

291 kcal Calories | 30 g Fat | 6 g Carbs | 9 g Proteins

Ingredients

- 2 tbsp of cocoa, Dutch processed
- 2 tbsp Monk Fruit sweetener
- 1 egg
- 2 drops of food color super red, it's optional
- 1/4 tsp of baking powder
- 1 tbsp of whipping cream (heavy)
- For Frosting
- 2 tbsp of Monk Fruit sweetener
- 2 tbsp of softened cream cheese at room temp
- 1/4 tsp of clear vanilla

Directions

1. Whisk the egg in a little bowl

2. Transfer the rest of the ingredients and blend until the mixture is creamy and smooth

3. Place half the mixture into a waffle maker then cook for about 2 1/2–3
minutes till it is cooked completely

4. Put the cream cheese, sweetener and vanilla in a separate, little bowl. Blend the frosting till all is fully mixed

5. Apply the frosting over the chaffle cake after bringing it to room tem- perature exactly

Pumpkin-cinnamon Churro Sticks

Servings: 2

Cooking Time: 14 Minutes

Ingredients:

- 3 tbsp coconut flour
- ¼ cup pumpkin puree
- 1 egg, beaten
- ½ cup finely grated mozzarella cheese
- 2 tbsp sugar-free maple syrup + more for serving
- 1 tsp baking powder
- 1 tsp vanilla extract
- ½ tsp pumpkin spice seasoning
- 1/8 tsp salt
- 1 tbsp cinnamon powder

Directions:

Preheat the waffle iron.

Mix all the ingredients in a medium bowl until well combined.

Open the iron and add half of the mixture. Close and cook until golden brown and crispy, 7 minutes.

Remove the chaffle onto a plate and make 1 more with the remaining batter.

Cut each chaffle into sticks, drizzle the top with more maple syrup and serve after.

Nutrition Info: Per Servings: Calories 219 | Fats 9.72g | Carbs 8.g | Net Carbs 4.34g | Protein 25.27g

Sharp Cheddar Chaffles

Servings: 2

Cooking Time: 10 Minutes

Ingredients:

*   1 organic egg, beaten
*   ½ cup sharp Cheddar cheese, shredded

Directions:

Preheat a mini waffle iron and then grease it.

In a small bowl, place the egg and cheese and stir to combine.

Place half of the mixture into preheated waffle iron and cook for about 5 minutes or until golden brown.

Repeat with the remaining mixture. Serve warm.

Nutrition Info:

Per Servings: Calories: 145 | Net Carb: 0.5g | Fat: 11 | Saturated Fat: 6.6g | Carbohydrates: 0.5g | Dietary Fiber: 0g Sugar: 0.3g | Protein: 9.8g

Put in the mayonnaise, bacon, and egg. to the chaffle

Low-Carb Chocolate Chip Vanilla Chaffles

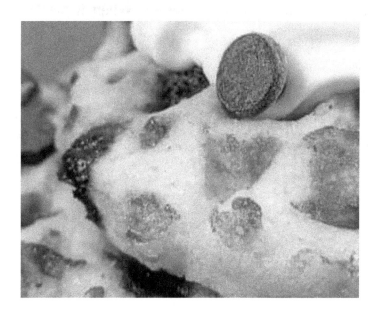

Servings: 1-2 Preparation Time: 1 min Nutrition Facts:

386 kcal calories | 28.1 g Fat |

8.2 g Carbs | 24.7 g Proteins

Ingredients

- 1/2 cup of pre-shredded or grated mozzarella

- 1 egg

- 1 tbsp granulated sugar substitute

- 1 tsp of vanilla extract

- 2 tbsp of almond meal or flour

- 1 tbsp of chocolate chips

Directions

Integrate your chosen components together in a bowl

Preheat your mini waffle processor. When it becomes hot, sprinkle with olive oil & spill half the mixture into the waffle maker

Cook for 2 to 4 min and then put it out and repeat

You must be capable of making two mini-chaffles each recipe

Topping, serve, as well as celebrate

SWEET CHAFFLE RECIPES

Keto Breakfast Chaffle Sandwich

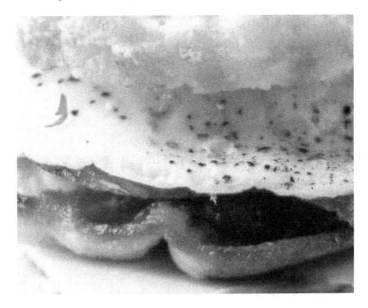

Servings: 1

Preparation time: 10 minutes Nutritional values:

346.6 kcal Calories | 27.9 g Fat | 1.2g Carbs | 22.5g Proteins

Ingredients

- 1 Large egg
- 1\2 of shredded cheese (cheddar)
- 2 tsp mayonnaise
- 1-2 pcs of bacon
- 1 egg

Directions

Heat up the mini waffle iron

Add the shredded cheese and the egg in a little bowl, whereas the waffle iron is heating

Pour half the batter onto the waffle maker and cook 3-4 minutes or until you want waffles close

Cook the bacon in a small saucepan until crispy nicely browned, then

set aside

Cook the egg to ideal doneness using the same tiny saucepan, add sea salt and pepper to fit

Club Sandwich Chaffle

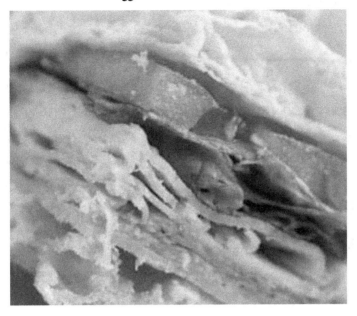

Servings: 1-2

Preparation time: 10 minutes Nutritional Values:

1078 kcal Calories | 86 g Fat | 12 g Carbs | 66 g Proteins

Ingredients

- 2 batches of chaffle simple recipe
- 2 strips of sugar-free bacon
- 2 Oz free of sugar sliced deli turkey
- 2 Oz sugar-free sliced deli ham
- 1 slice of cheese (cheddar)
- 1 tomato slice
- 3 lettuce leaves
- 1 tbsp mayonnaise free of sugar

Directions

Cook the chaffles and put aside, as instructed. Cover to keep warm Cook the Bacon using your chosen (oven/microwave/stovetop) cook- ing process. By putting them in the microwave, sealed, keep it basic for around 2-3 minutes (based on how crispy you want it and the brand). When cooked, move to a lined sheet of paper towel

Make your sandwich, start the club sandwich with one chaffle and com- plete with the tomato and the lettuce. Add the other chaffle and the cheese, ham, turkey and Bacon on top. Smear the final chaffle with mayo, then put it on top of the sandwich Enjoy it right away

Keto Chaffle (Cheese Waffle) Plus Omad Sandwich

Servings: 1

Preparation time: 5 minutes Nutritional Values:

WAFFLE:

458 kcal Calories | 33.4g Fat | 3.5g Carbs | 26.7g Proteins

SANDWICH:

1168 kcal Calories | 84.2g Fat | 8.7g Carbs | 99.4g Proteins

Ingredients WAFFLE

- 3/4 cup (75 g) shredded cheese (any of your choice)
- 1 medium-sized egg
- 1 tsp husk of psyllium
- salt / pepper
- Hot sauce (Optional) SANDWICH
- 4 bacon strips
- 4 ham slices
- 4 prosciutto slices
- 5-6 salami slices
- 5-6 small pepperoni slices
- Mustard
- Mayonnaise

Directions

Whisk the egg, cheese, salt, pepper, psyllium husk together in a bowl,

and additional hot sauce

Keep the waffle maker to heat until the batter is uniformly poured into the waffle pan

Cook 2-3 minutes or more based on how crispy you like it to be

Carry it out and eat the sandwich as is or top with delicious ingredients, fat-filled dinner

Cheesy Chaffle Sandwich's with Avocado and Bacon

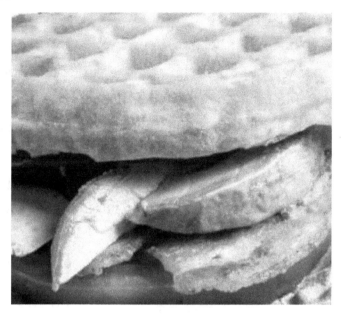

Servings: 1-2

Preparation time: 25 minutes Nutritional Values:

259 kcal Calories | 20.1 g Fat | 6.8 g Carbs | 14 g Proteins

Ingredients

- 10 eggs
- 1 1/2 cups of shredded cheddar cheese
- 2 center cut slices of bacon, cooked and crumbled
- ½ tsp of ground pepper
- 2 small, sliced avocados
- 2 little tomatoes, in slices
- 4 large lettuce leaves, torn into 3 "parts

Directions

In a large bowl, whisk the eggs until smooth. Stir in cheese and chopped bacon and pepper

Preheat a 7-inch (not Belgian) round waffle iron; top it with cooking spray. Pour approximately 2/3 cup of the beaten egg into the waffle iron. Cook 4 to 5 minutes till the eggs are set and light golden brown. Repeat with cooking spray and the residual mixture of eggs (making a total of 4 chaffles)

Split each of the chaffles into pieces. Top half of the quarters even with slices of avocado, tomato slices and lettuce. Also, top the remaining quarters of the chaffle

Mozzarellas & Psyllium Husk Chaffles

Servings: 2

Cooking Time: 8 Minutes

Ingredients:

- ½ cup Mozzarella cheese, shredded
- 1 large organic egg, beaten
- 2 tablespoons blanched almond flour
- ½ teaspoon Psyllium husk powder
- ¼ teaspoon organic baking powder

Directions:

Preheat a mini waffle iron and then grease it.

In a bowl, place all the ingredients and beat until well combined.

Place half of the mixture into preheated waffle iron and cook for about 4 minutes or until golden brown.

Repeat with the remaining mixture. Serve warm.

Nutrition Info:

Per Servings: Calories: 101 | Net Carb: 1 | Fat: 7.1g |
Saturated Fat: 1.8g | Carbohydrates: 2.9g | Dietary Fiber: 1.3g
Sugar: 0.2g | Protein: 6.7g

Chocolate & Almond Chaffle

Servings: 3

Cooking Time: 12 Minutes

Ingredients:

- 1 egg
- ¼ cup mozzarella cheese, shredded
- 1 oz. cream cheese
- 2 teaspoons sweetener
- 1 teaspoon vanilla
- 2 tablespoons cocoa powder
- 1 teaspoon baking powder
- 2 tablespoons almonds, chopped
- 4 tablespoons almond flour

Directions:

Blend all the ingredients in a bowl while the waffle maker is preheating. Pour some of the mixture into the waffle maker. Close and cook for 4 minutes.

Transfer the chaffle to a plate. Let cool for 2 minutes. Repeat steps using the remaining mixture.

Nutrition Info: Calories 1 | Total Fat 13.1g | Saturated Fat 5g | Cholesterol 99mg | Sodium 99mg | Potassium 481mg Total Carbohydrate 9.1g | Dietary Fiber 3.8g | Protein 7.8g Total Sugars 0.8g

Low Carb Keto Chaffle Sandwich

Servings: 1-2

Preparation time: 10 minutes

Nutritional Values: 320 kcal Calories | 24g Fat | 5g Carbs | 21g Proteins

Ingredients

- 10 tbsp parmesan shredded cheese
- 1 cup of mozzarella shredded
- 2 slices of bacon (chopped)
- 1/4 tsp dry oregano
- 1 heaping tbsp of birch benders pancake mix (can be substituted for gf flour or desired mixture)
- 2 chickens 2 eggs
- Mayo
- 2 tiny or 1 large, thinly cut tomato
- Salt and pepper to fit

Directions

Put the egg, oregano, mozzarella cheese pancake mixture and salt and pepper into a food processor. Pulse blend until complete. Should just take a few steps

Add bacon and pulse in the mixture until bacon is uniformly dispersed Put 1 tbsp of parmesan on the waffle maker bottom. 1 Heaping waffle mixture spoonful and 1 tbsp parmesan on top. Cover the waffle maker and finish cooking till golden brown. Repeat until the entire mix is used. It can yield about five mini waffles

Apply mayo on the waffle side. Add sliced tomato, salt and pepper to taste. Attach 2nd waffle to the end, and you've got a tomato sammie chaffle

Keto Snickerdoodle Chaffles

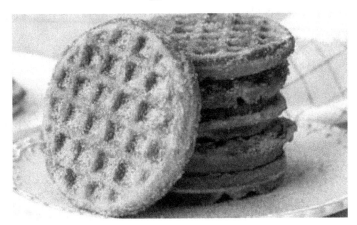

Servings: 1

Preparation time: 15 minutes Nutritional values:

186 kcal Calories | 15.5 g Fat | 3.2 g Carbs | 8.4 g Proteins

Ingredients Waffles:

- 1 egg, large
- 1/2 cup of crushed mozzarella (low-moisture)
- 1/4 cup of almond flour
- 1/8 tsp of baking powder, gluten-free
- 3 tbsp of low-carb granulated sweeteners like swerve or eryth-ritol

Topping

- 1 1/2 tbsp of unsalted butter, melted
- 1 tsp of cinnamon
- 3 tbsp of low-carb granulated sweeteners like swerve or eryth-ritol

Directions

1.   For the waffles, measure all the ingredients. Preheat your waffle machine

2.   You may either add all of the components in a medium bowl then mix them until incorporated or blend them together. Put the mozzarella, eggs, almond flour & baking powder in a food processor or blender for this

3. Insert the sweetener then mix in. Blending remains optional but strongly encouraged

4.   To form 3 small chaffles, pour a third of the mixture into the preheated waffle maker

5.   Cover the maker then cook for three to four mins. Keep a close eye on the mixture if it overflows

6.   Lift the lid once ready, and allow it to cool down for a little bit. Using a spatula to move the chaffle softly onto a cooling tray

7.   Repeat the procedure for the batter, which is remaining. When they're hot, the chaffles will be fluffy but would crisp up when they're finally chill

Strawberries and Cream Keto Chaffles

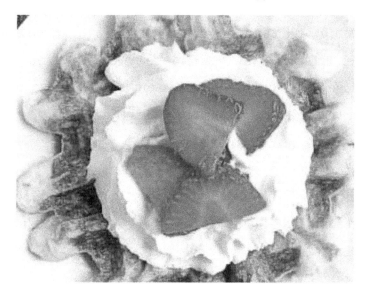

Servings: 1-2

Preparation Time: 25 min Nutritional Values:

189 kcal Calories | 14.3 g Fat | 5.2 g Carbs | 10 g Proteins

Ingredients

- 3 ounces of cream cheese
- 2 cups of mozzarella cheese, shredded
- 2 eggs, whipped
- 1/2 cup of almond flour
- 2 tsp of baking powder
- Eight strawberries
- A cup of whipped cream i.e., canister- two tbsp per waffle
- 1 tbsp of confectioner's sweetener, swerve

Directions

Put the mozzarella and the cream cheese to a microwave bowl and then cook for 1 min. Mix properly, then proceed to the next stage, if all of the cheese is melted. Or else cook for another 30 seconds and then combine properly

Beat the eggs in some other bowl, then add baking powder, almond flour and 3 tbsp swerve sweetener

Combine the mixture of cream cheese with the mixture of almond flour then blend properly, now add in Two chopped strawberries. Put it in the fridge for 20 min

Meanwhile, cut the leftover strawberries and apply Swerve's one table- spoon. Mix properly and set it aside or cold

Then pull the batter out from the refrigerator, after 20 min. Heat up the waffle iron, then go on for that so, if it has to be greased

Pick 1/4 cup of mix and transfer to the hot iron, to the middle. Ensure the waffles are tiny so that they'll be easy to bring out from the waffle maker Whenever it's prepared, move to a plate and then let it be cool before adding strawberries and whipped cream

Blt Chaffle Sandwich

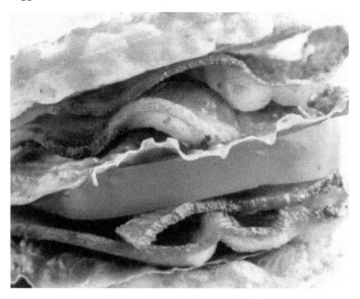

Servings: 2

Preparation time: 10 minutes Nutritional values:

183 kcal Calories | 13.9 g Fat |

1.4 g Carbs | 10.8 g Proteins

Ingredients for chaffle

- 1/2 cup, shredded mozzarella
- 1 egg
- 1 tbsp of green onion, chopped
- 1/2 tsp Seasoning (Italian)

Ingredients for Sandwich

- Pre-cooked bacon
- Lettuce

- Tomato, in slices
- 1 tbs of mayo

Directions

Heat up the mini-waffle maker Whip the egg in a little bowl Add the cheese, seasonings and onion to blend. Mix until it's fully set in In the mini waffle maker, place half the batter and cook for 4 minutes

If you want a crunchy crust, apply a teaspoon of grated cheese to the mini waffle iron before adding the batter for 30 seconds. Extra cheese will create the best crust on the outside

Following the completion of the first chaffle, add the rest batter to the waffle maker and cook for 4 minutes

Fill your sandwich with the mayo, Bacon, lettuce, and tomato

Garlic Bread Chaffle

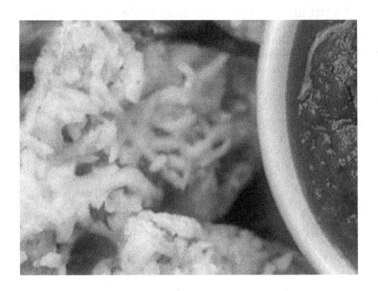

Serving: 2

Preparation time: 5 minutes Nutritional Value:

186 kcal Calories | 14 g Fat | 3 g Carbs| 10 g Proteins

Ingredients

- 1 large egg
- 1/2 cup of mozzarella, finely shredded
- 1 tsp of coconut flour
- ¼ tsp of baking powder
- 1/2 tsp of garlic powder
- 1 tbsp of melted butter
- 1/4 tsp of garlic salt
- 2 tbsp of Parmesan
- 1 tsp of finely chopped parsley

Directions

Plugin, to preheat your waffle maker. Set Oven temperature to 375F and preheat

In a mixing bowl, add the mozzarella, egg, coconut flour, garlic powder and baking powder and stir well to blend

Put half the batter in the waffle iron, then cook about 3 min or till the steam has ended. On a baking sheet, put the prepared chaffle

With the leftover batter of the chaffle, repeat the same steps

Mix garlic salt and butter together, then over the chaffles, brush it Sprinkle the Parmesan on the chaffles

Put the pan, 5 min in the oven to the cheese to be melt Scatter the parsley over it prior to serving

Notes

The garlic salt renders them mildly salty-if you're watching salt, feel free to add in freshly chopped garlic or even garlic powder.

Keto Taco Chaffles

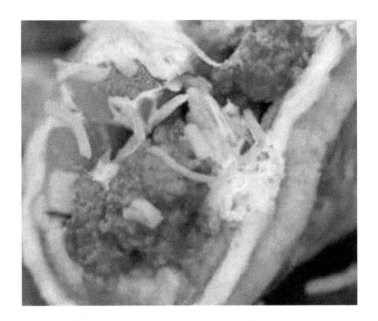

Servings: 3-4

Preparation time: 5 minutes Nutritional Values:

258 kcal Calories | 19 g Fat | 4 g Carbs | 18 g Proteins

Ingredients

- 1 egg white
- 1/4 cup of shredded Monterey jack cheese, (packed firmly)
- 1/4 cup of shredded sharp cheddar cheese, (packed firmly)
- 3/4 tsp of water
- 1 tsp of coconut flour
- 1/4 tsp of baking powder
- 1/8 tsp of chili powder
- 1 pinch salt

Directions

Plugin the wall, the Mini Waffle Maker and lightly grease it once it is warm

Incorporate all the components in a bowl and mix well to combine them Pour half of the mixture on the maker and then shut the lid
Setup a 4-min timer, and thus do not remove the cover till the cooking duration is finished

If you do so, the taco chaffle will appear like it is not set up completely, but it would

Before you open the lid, you get to just let it prepare the whole 4 min Put the taco shell out from the iron as well as set aside. Repeat the same procedure for the remaining portion of the chaffle batter

Switch a muffin pan over and place the taco chaffle between cups to create a taco shell. Let to set it for a couple of minutes

Keto Blueberry Chaffle

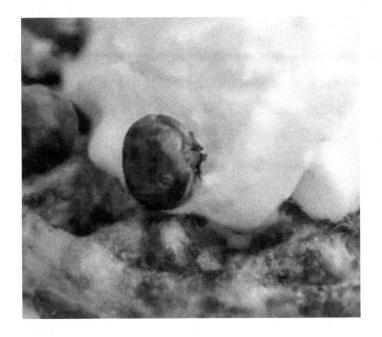

Servings: 1-2

Preparation Time: 3 minutes Nutritional Value:

116 kcal Calories | 8 g Fat | 3 g Carbs | 8 g Proteins

Ingredients

- 1 cup mozzarella cheese
- 2 tbsp of almond flour
- 1 tsp of baking powder
- 2 eggs
- 1 tsp of cinnamon
- 2 tsp of swerve
- 3 tbsp of blueberries

Directions

Preheat your waffle maker

Put the almond flour, mozzarella cheese, baking powder, cinnamon, eggs, swerve & blueberries into a mixing bowl. Stir properly enough that the ingredients blend well

Sprinkle non-stick spray on the waffle maker

Insert less than one fourth a cup of keto blueberry waffle mixture

Shut the lid, then for 3-5 min, cook the chaffle. Assess it at 3 min to see whether it's brown & crispy. Whether it isn't or if it sticks to the waffle maker's top, shut the cover then cook for 1 to 2 min

Represent with a light sprinkling of swerve or keto syrup

CPSIA information can be obtained
at www.ICGtesting.com
Printed in the USA
LVHW100741190421
684817LV00022B/133

9 781914 516245